LIVING A LENGTHY LIFE:

NUTRITION GUIDES TO LIVING LONGER

Len Glover

Copyright

Copyright © Len Glover. All rights reserved.

Contents

- **Food Sources to Eat Consistently for Better Cerebrum Wellbeing**
- **Hints to work on your Memory**
- **Methods for Losing Gut Fat and Carry on with a Better Life**
- **Recuperating FOOD Fundamentals THAT Advance Injury Mending**

Introduction

Way of life changes, including a sound eating routine, actual activity, and mental activity could assume a significant part in the counteraction of Alzheimer's illness. A Mediterranean eating regimen may decrease the hazard of Alzheimer's, yet may likewise lessen mortality from the illness. Various leafy foods seem to help different mental spaces of the cerebrum, so both assortment and amount in the eating routine are significant. More noteworthy foods grown from the ground utilization have been connected with lower paces of dementia and Alzheimer's sickness. The utilization of blueberries and strawberries is related to postponed mental maturing by as much as 2.5 years. Ellagic corrosive might assume a part in the capacity of berries to forestall age-related mental deterioration, yet its retention is impeded by dairy.

The connection between tofu and dementia might be connected with formaldehyde defilement. Squeezed apples didn't seem to increment mental execution in Alzheimer's patients, even though in a petri dish, squeezed apple and ginger seemed to further develop nerve cell endurance. In any case, it has been found that the people who drink foods grown from ground juices had a 76% lower chance of fostering Alzheimer's, conceivably due to phytonutrient content. Saffron, when contrasted with Aricept, a main medication in the treatment of Alzheimer's, was found to work similarly too without the secondary effects (see likewise here). While populaces eating more turmeric have a lower rate of Alzheimer's, this might be because of their lower utilization of meat, which is likewise useful for Parkinson's sickness. Nonetheless, turmeric, yet not curcumin supplements, was found to ease Alzheimer patients' side effects. Espresso may likewise decrease the gamble of Parkinson's and Alzheimer's. On the other hand, there is little proof that coconut oil assists with Alzheimer's sickness. Aluminum is added to handle cheddar and might be connected with neurodegenerative illnesses like Alzheimer's. Essentially, iron collection in the cerebrum is by and large progressively connected to neurological illnesses like Alzheimer's, mycotoxins (viewed as generally in chicken) may expand the gamble of fostering Alzheimer's sickness, and BMAA, a neurotoxin found in fish may likewise be connected with higher paces of neurodegenerative infection. Besides, there's been a suggestion that individuals with a family background of neurodegenerative infections ought to keep away from milk. Harmful material in the food supply might assist with making sense of the connection between dairy utilization and Parkinson's sickness (see likewise here). Skim milk has been found to have particularly elevated degrees of chemicals. There might be a basic, modest, painless test for the location of Alzheimer's illness.

The utilization of methylmercury can bring about microcephaly, impeded comprehension, and deferred cerebrum nerve correspondence in babies, babies, and youngsters. Mercury tainting has additionally been connected to bringing down intelligence levels and mind harm in the offspring of moms who ingest mercury while pregnant. Ladies might need to stay away from contaminated fish utilization for a year before they get pregnant as well as during pregnancy. Methyl mercury is tracked down in fish and fish (see here, here, and). Ayurvedic prescriptions have likewise been viewed as sullied with mercury and lead. Arsenic is taken care of by chickens and might be connected with neuropathy as well as neurocognitive deficiencies in youngsters. Getting bitewing or all-encompassing X-beams at the dental specialist might be related to an expanded gamble of meningioma, the most widely recognized kind of mind cancer. Drying out may debilitate mental capabilities.

Causes of Some Major Diseases

Pork tapeworm hatchlings attacking the mind is one of the most well-known reasons for epilepsy and may present as headaches or persistent pressure migraines.

The mind parasite toxoplasma is tracked down in sheep; 10% of Americans are right now contaminated with this parasite. There are likewise transient skin worms from sushi utilization that might get into the cerebrum.

Neurotoxic synthetic compounds in chicken, including beta-carboline alkaloids, may likewise make sense of the connection between meat utilization and the normal neurological problem fundamental quake. There are neurotoxins in fish that can't be killed with cooking and can cause peculiar responses (like hot feels like cool, cold feels hot).

Likewise, domoic corrosive, found in fish, has been found to cause a surprising type of amnesia.

Ibuprofen normally found in plants might make sense of the presence of headache medicine in the circulation system of veggie lovers. The omega-3 unsaturated fats our cerebrum needs for ideal well-being (both long and short-chain) can be acquired from plant sources.

Blue-green growth can create neurotoxins and ought to be itwawayom. Mental shortfalls might be an early indication of B12 lack, which is more continuous in veggie lovers and vegans than omnivores.

What Might Assist You with Becoming Effective?

I have been doing this quick for quite a long time on and off and I have attempted a few eating times. What I found that turns out best for me was to skip breakfast and eat my most memorable feast at noon and last dinner at 8 pm. This permits me to eat supper with loved ones. My most memorable feast will in general be weighty versus my last dinner is lighter. You have an 8-hour window. Do what works for you.

Be careful, it will require several days for your body to change. This will rely upon your way of life preceding fasting. Assuming that you've been eating leafy foods. It may not affect the off chance that you have not. Your body will require time to change to the new eating system.

Plan out your feasts ahead of time. You might need to go similarly as have a few feasts as of now prepared. Keep lots of water with you. Assuming that you drink espresso, keep it dark with no additional items in it. This will assist you with avoiding the features going off your arrangement.

Eat a lot of food. Getting every one of your supplements by eating leafy foods is vital. This will assist with lessening any desires. Assuming you are working out, protein powders might be ideal to add to your smoothies.

For this quick natural leafy foods are best. No canned natural products or vegetables. You can have new spices and flavors. Natural teas come exceptionally convenient, particularly after your last feast.

Here are some smoothie recipes I have utilized before. You can get innovative with them and think of your adaptation.

What to eat to live lengthily

The five dietary patterns that can expand your life, as per an enrolled dietitian.

The vast majority need to carry on with a more drawn-out life. Be that as it may, the objective of life span is likewise to carry on with a superior life, with work on mental and actual health and the capacity to be dynamic and free. In my years as an enlisted dietitian, I've seen a lot of individuals in their 70s, 80s, and past who are more grounded than people a portion of their age.

While hereditary qualities truly do assume a part, way of life is a huge component, and sustenance is a major piece of the riddle. A 2016 survey of the writing distributed in the diary Resistance and Maturing refers to concentrates on that propose that 25% of one's life is not entirely set in stone by hereditary qualities the rest is impacted by way of life.

The following are five dietary patterns to embrace to build your possibilities, broaden your life and partake in every year with energy.

1. <u>Eat Your Veggies and Organic Product</u>

I realize you hear this one a great deal, however eating more produce is genuinely quite possibly of the most significant and effective propensity you can embrace. Sadly, most Americans are off track of the imprint. As per the Habitats for Infectious Prevention and Counteraction (CDC), somewhere around one out of 10 U.S. grown-ups eats an adequate number of veggies and organic products. Simply 10% hit the prescribed few day-to-day cups of veggies, and 12% arrive at the everyday objects of one-and-a-half to two cups of natural product.

As well as increasing your supplement consumption, arriving at those essentials might add a very long time to your life. A 2017 meta-examination distributed in the Worldwide Diary of The study of disease transmission observed that higher utilization of leafy foods is related to a lower chance of mortality from all causes, including coronary illness and malignant growth. Hold back nothing five servings per day. More is fine, however, in some exploration, the gamble of death didn't lessen further past this sum.

2. <u>Step-by-step instructions to Eat More Products of the soil</u>

Work in two cups of foods grown from the ground cups of veggies every day, with one cup being about the size of a tennis ball. A few hints: Have a go at getting into a daily schedule of integrating a cup of organic product into each morning meal and a second as a component of a day-to-day nibble. Integrate one cup of veggies at lunch and two at supper. Or on the other hand, consolidate them. A smoothie made with a small bunch of greens and a cup of frozen berries takes out two. You can likewise add new natural products, such as cut apples or orange cuts, to entrée servings of mixed greens and pan-fried food recipes.

3. <u>Go crazy for Nuts and Nut Spreads</u>

Nuts are sustenance forces to be reckoned with. They give fortifying fat, plant protein, fiber, cancer prevention agents, nutrients, and key minerals, similar to potassium and magnesium. It's no big surprise they're connected to life augmentation.

As indicated by the Public Heart, Lung, and Blood Foundation (NHLBI), metabolic disorder, otherwise known as insulin obstruction condition, is a gathering of conditions that increment an individual's gamble of coronary illness, diabetes, and stroke.

A 2020 randomized preliminary that was important for a bigger report distributed in The Diary of Sustenance followed 5,800 people with metabolic conditions for a year. Results propose that as nut utilization expanded, certain markers for metabolic conditions diminished. These markers incorporate midsection periphery, fatty substance levels, systolic circulatory strain, weight, and BMI. HDL, the great cholesterol, likewise expanded in ladies engaged with the review (however not the men).

4. <u>Step-by-step instructions to Eat More Nuts</u>

An ounce of nuts is about a quarter cup, however, two tablespoons of nut spread likewise consider a serving. Whip nut margarine into your smoothie, mix it into oats, or use it as a plunge for a new natural product or celery. Add nuts to plates of mixed greens, cooked veggies, and pan-fried food recipes, or eat them with no guarantees. Squashed nuts additionally make an incredible choice for bread pieces to cover fish or embellishment dishes like crushed cauliflower or lentil soup. Baking with nut flours or involving them in flapjacks is one more extraordinary method for increasing your admission.

5. <u>Eat More Without Meat Feasts</u>

Meatless Mondays have been a thing for quite a long time. That is phenomenal, however, for a life span, you ought to fabricate plant-based dinners into your eating routine over one day seven days.

In a 2016 article in the American Diary of Way of Life Medication, scientists depict five regions in existence where individuals reside the longest, and best reside. Considered

Blue Zones, these locales are tracked down in exceptionally different regions, from Okinawa, Japan to Ikaria, Greece. One shared trait they share is the utilization of essentially plant-based abstains from food. Beans and lentils are foundations, and meat is eaten normally around five times each month in three-to four-ounce segments — about the size of a deck of cards.

The main Blue Zone in the US is in Loma Linda, California, which has the most elevated grouping of Seventh-Day Adventists. By and large, 10 years longer than their North American partners.

For instance, a recent report distributed in JAMA Inside Medication took a gander at the north of 73,000 Seventh-Day Adventist people and viewed that when contrasted with omnivores, the individuals who stayed with a veggie lover diet had a fundamentally lower by and large mortality risk. This included veggie lovers, lacto-ovo vegans (who in all actuality do eat dairy and eggs), and pisco vegans (who do eat fish). A 2019 subsequent review to 2013 one, distributed in the Diary of Healthful Science, saw that when contrasted with the eating regimen of non-vegans, veggie lovers consuming fewer calories were related to fundamentally lower levels of cardiovascular sickness risk factors.

What's more, in a recent report in PLOS Medication, specialists took a gander at what food decisions mean for the future. They verified that the biggest additions in life span could be made by "eating more vegetables, entire grains and nuts, and less red and handled meat."

The most effective method to Eat Less Meat

To receive the rewards, trade the meat in dinners for beats, the umbrella term for beans, lentils, peas, and chickpeas. Settle on lentil or dark bean soup as an afterthought as opposed to adding chicken to a serving of mixed greens. Utilize dark-peered peas in a sautéed food instead of meat, and nibble on veggies with hummus rather than jerky. Investigate ethnic cafés in your space that proposition beat-based dishes, similar to Indian chickpea curry and Ethiopian lentil stew.

Eat Like a Mediterranean

With regards to life span, it's the general eating design, as opposed to one food or nutrition type, that is critical. A Mediterranean eating regimen stays one of the best quality levels for living longer and more refreshingly. This example is described by a high admission of leafy foods; entire grains; beats; empowering fats from nuts, olive oil, and avocado; and spices and flavors. It incorporates fish a couple of times each week. The Mediterranean eating regimen additionally incorporates moderate utilization of dairy, eggs, and wine and restricts the admission of meat and desserts.

One proportion of life span frequently referred to in the examination at the cell level is telomere length. More or less, telomeres are covers found at the closures of chromosomes that safeguard DNA. At the point when they become too short, a cell ages significantly or is broken. To this end, more limited telomeres are related to a lower future and an expanded gamble of creating constant illnesses. Research distributed in 2017 in the diary Oncotarget recommends that more prominent adherence to a Mediterranean eating routine is connected to life span through keeping up with longer telomere length. A similar report showed that for every one-point increase in the Mediterranean eating routine score (which estimates adherence to the eating routine), the gamble of death from any reason drops by 4 to 7%.

The most effective method to Eat a Mediterranean Eating routine

To mediterranean-ize your dinners, supplant spread with nut margarine or avocado on toast and exchange it for additional virgin olive oil to sauté vegetables. Nibble on new natural products with nuts, olives, or cooked chickpeas, and keep feasts straightforward. A reasonable Prescription eating regimen supper might comprise fish served over a bed of greens thrown in additional virgin olive oil with a side of cooked potatoes or quinoa and a glass of pinot noir.

Taste Green Tea

I like to allude to green tea as a precautionary medication in a mug. Various examinations have connected it to a lower chance of coronary illness, malignant growth, type 2 diabetes, Alzheimer's, and corpulence. In a 2022 survey of the writing distributed in the diary Supplements, scientists found that those with the most noteworthy green tea consumption had lower paces of cardiovascular sickness, as well as a lower hazard of passing on from coronary illness and stroke. And keeping in mind that it can't be said conclusively that drinking green tea will make you live longer, there are by all accounts a few relationships between life span and green tea consumption.

The most effective method to Drink More Green Tea

As well as tasting, you can involve green tea as the fluid in smoothies, oats, or short-term oats, or to steam veggies or entire grain rice. It can likewise be integrated into soups, stews, sauces, and marinades. Matcha, a powdered type of green tea, can likewise be utilized in drinks and recipes. Simply make certain to remove all caffeine no less than six hours before sleep time so you will not disturb your rest length or quality.

A Fast Survey

To the extent that what not to do, it's the standard suspects. Try not to indulge or polish off a lot of sugar, handled food varieties, meat, or liquor. Fortunately, the defensive food varieties above can without much of a stretch dislodge maturing prompting food varieties. Go after an apple with almond margarine instead of handled treats, and supplant soft drinks with green tea. All in all, attention to what to eat, and you'll normally control your admission of food sources to keep away from. That is significant because, for a lifespan, consistency is critical. A long stretch eating routine backings a long, solid life!

Food assortments associated with better mental capacity

In like manner, as there is no spellbound pill to frustrate mental disintegrating, no single area of strength for all food can guarantee a sharp cerebrum as you age. Nutritionists stress that the fundamental strategy is to follow a strong dietary model that integrates a lot of regular items, vegetables, vegetables, and whole grains. Try to get protein from plant sources and fish and pick sound fats, like olive oil or canola, instead of soaked fats.

Research shows that the best mind food combinations are the very ones that safeguard your heart and veins, incorporating the going with Green, verdant vegetables.

Research suggests these plant-based food assortments could help with moving back mental corruption.

Oily fish. Smooth fish are plentiful wellsprings of omega-3 unsaturated fats, strong unsaturated fats that have been connected with slashed blood levels of beta-amyloid the protein that plans to hurt packs in the cerebrums of individuals with Alzheimer's sickness. Attempt to eat fish something like two times reliably, besides pick assortments that are low in mercury, like salmon, cod, canned light fish, and pollack.

Berries, Flavonoids, the ordinary plant colors that give berries their marvelous colors, moreover help with additional creating memory research shows.

Tea and espresso, The caffeine in your morning mug of espresso or tea could offer something past blazing fixation support. In a new report dispersed in The Journal of Sustenance, individuals with higher caffeine use scored better on preliminaries of mental capacity. Caffeine could in like manner help with solidifying new memories, as shown by different assessments. Inspectors at Johns Hopkins School mentioned individuals focus on a progression of pictures and thereafter take either a phony treatment or a 200-milligram caffeine tablet. More people from the caffeine bundle had the choice to precisely perceive the photos on the following day.

Walnuts. Nuts are incredible wellsprings of protein and sound fats, and one sort of nut explicitly could moreover additionally foster memory. A new report from UCLA associated higher walnut use with additional created mental grades. Includes calories are rich in ALA and other omega-3 unsaturated fats have been associated with a cut-down heartbeat and cleaner veins. That is perfect for both the heart and frontal cortex cerebrum.

55

The job of a plant-based diet in switching sickness

Changing to a plant-based diet can have a larger number of advantages than simply weight reduction. Truth be told, remembering all the more entire food varieties and greens for your eating routine can assist with turning around a few constant illnesses and assume a significant part in sickness counteraction.

Something worth mulling over

While organizing your eating regimen, you need to ponder food varieties that are plentiful in nutrients and minerals. These food things can assist with bringing down your pulse and terrible cholesterol, in this way assisting with forestalling or overseeing illnesses like diabetes and coronary illness.

Visiting a way-of-life medication expert can assist you with refocusing while beginning your new eating regimen. The person will want to make a way of life plan that works for him or them and survey your family ancestry to best figure out what illnesses he ought to be proactive in forestall.

Food sources to incorporate

Your plant-based diet ought to incorporate non-boring vegetables, vegetables, and new foods grown from the ground. These are infection-battling food varieties that are not difficult to integrate into your day-to-day feasts.

Great vegetable decisions incorporate broccoli, kale, cabbage, Brussels sprouts, mushrooms, onions, and peppers. If all else fails, practice environmental awareness and verdant.

For energy, you ought to likewise eat vegetables as a wellspring of carbs. These incorporate beans, lentils, peas, and different food varieties plentiful in B-bunch nutrients. Routinely eating vegetables can assist with diminishing your gamble of creating diabetes and colon disease.

Nuts likewise have numerous medical advantages. They furnish the body with solid fat and have mitigating impacts that can bring down your possibility of creating cardiovascular illness and coronary illness.

In conclusion, new natural products like berries, citrus, and tomatoes function as cell reinforcements and can assist with forestalling coronary illness and a few malignant growths.

Food sources to stay away from

Numerous food varieties ought to be kept away from because of their part in adding to stoutness, coronary illness, diabetes, and other persistent illnesses. The primary offenders as a rule incorporate an overabundance of salt, sugar, immersed fat, trans, fat,t, and straightforward carbs. Models are broiled food sources like French fries and potato chips, and sweet beverages like pop and feasts focused on bread, similar to pizza and pasta.

Rather than eating low-quality food and sweet tidbits, settle on plant-based things that are filling, similar to beans or vegetables. If you are truly longing for a sweet treat, eat a little piece of natural product or dim chocolate.

If you are keen on embracing a plant-based diet, visit a way-of-life medication expert for more data.

Step-by-step instructions to Dispose of Sicknesses Normally: A Manual for Restorative Opportunity

There is a ton of talk nowadays about normal cures and how to dispose of sicknesses normally. For some individuals, this is an appealing choice, as it permits them to assume command over their well-being and keeps away from the results of ordinary prescriptions. Infections can be unquestionably crippling and life-changing. However, imagine a scenario where there were regular ways of disposing of them without the utilization of medications or medical procedures. This guide will tell you the best way to turn out to be liberated from the shackles of customary medication. With this data, you'll have the option to assume command over your well-being and prosperity.

Support YOUR Safe Framework

The initial step to disposing of sicknesses normally is to support your invulnerable framework. You can do this by eating a sound eating routine, getting sufficient activity, and getting a lot of rest. Also, you can take supplements that assist to work on your safe framework. A few extraordinary choices incorporate L-ascorbic acid and garlic.

Spices

One more incredible method for disposing of infections normally is to ward them off with spices and other regular cures. There are a wide range of spices that have strong restorative properties. Probably the best ones for battling infection incorporate ginger, turmeric, oregano, and basil. You can involve these spices in teas, colors, or containers. They can likewise be added to food varieties or taken as enhancements.

Practice Great Cleanliness

As well as supporting your safe framework and fending off illnesses with spices, you can likewise keep them from occurring in any case. Perhaps the most ideal way to do this is to rehearse great cleanliness. This implies cleaning up consistently, staying away from close contact with individuals who are wiped out, and sanitizing surfaces that could be tainted. You ought to likewise receive an immunization shot against normal infections like flu and measles.

Way of life Adjustment

Many illnesses plague individuals from one side of the planet to the other. While some are effectively treatable, others can be persistent and lethal. However, consider the possibility that there was a method for disposing of sicknesses through naturopathy therapy, without costly prescriptions or therapies. Researchers are uncovering increasingly more proof that way of life adjustment is one of the most mind-blowing ways of remaining sound and illness free. By rolling out little improvements to your day-to-day daily schedule, including eating a sound eating regimen, getting standard activity, and keeping away from unfortunate things to do, you can keep your body working at its ideal and assist with keeping illness from grabbing hold.

Even though we have zeroed in on illness avoidance here, it is essential to recollect that there are numerous ways of freeing yourself of sicknesses normally. If you are searching for a more all-along-hauling and long-haul arrangement, consider attempting a portion of the strategies we've illustrated. Not exclusively will this work on your well-being, but, it might likewise assist with lessening your reliance on drugs. We expect that you will track down these tips accommodating in your excursion to better well-being. Assuming that you would like more data or have any inquiries, kindly feel free to Nirvana Naturopathy. We are here to assist you with carrying on with an illness-free life normally

Solid Way of Life

The mind is a vital organ. It's the control focus of your body and permits you to move, think, feel, and inhale and that's just the beginning. Since the mind has such a challenging task, we genuinely should furnish it with an overflow of fuel and supplements to help it capability appropriately and remain sound. The food sources we eat assume an enormous part in the construction and soundness of our cerebrums. A recent report distributed in General Wellbeing Sustenance showed that food varieties plentiful in nutrients, minerals, cell reinforcements, flavonols, polyphenols, and omega-3 unsaturated fats can assist with safeguarding your mind.

They can assist with further developing memory, fixation, and in general mental well-being.

Food Sources to Eat Consistently for Better Cerebrum Wellbeing

1. Salad Greens

Mixed greens, like kale and spinach, are loaded with supplements, including vitamin K, beta carotene (a forerunner to vitamin A), folate, and vitamin E. Vitamin E is a cell reinforcement that safeguards the cells from free extreme harm and has been connected to forestalling mental deterioration in the maturing populace. Vitamin K and beta carotene have likewise been connected to further developing mind well-being by assisting with forestalling cognitive decline and further developing insight. You can take a stab at adding a small bunch of greens while setting up a smoothie or adding a serving of greens to your #1 goulash recipe.

2. Sheep

Is it true that you love sheep? Assuming this is the case, you might be shocked to realize that sheep have been connected to advantages like long-haul discernment. As per a recent report distributed in the Diary of Alzheimer's Sickness, week after week utilization of sheep, but not other red meats, was related to working on long-haul comprehension. The 10-year concentrate on noted upgrades in liquid knowledge scores in people who polished off specific food sources, including sheep. Sheep is delivered in each state in the U.S. also, accessible all year, which makes it simple to add it to your eating regimen.

Have a go at adding sheep to your number one stew recipe or cooking it on the barbecue.

3. <u>Eggs</u>

Eggs are one of the most well-known breakfast food sources and for good explanation. They are cheap and offer a large group of medical advantages, particularly for cerebrum well-being. A recent report distributed in The American Diary of Clinical Nourishment found that customary utilization of eggs has been related with worked on mental execution in grown-ups. Choline has been related to decreasing bitterness and promoting mind qualification, such as keeping up with memory and correspondence between synapses.

Even though eggs are regularly served at breakfast, you can appreciate them at any dinner. Take a stab at utilizing eggs to make an exquisite supper quiche or a spectacular velvety custard for dessert.

4. <u>Salmon</u>

Salmon is normally known as an extraordinary wellspring of protein, however, did you have at least some idea that it is likewise perfect for mental well-being? Greasy fish like salmon is high in omega-3 unsaturated fats, which are basic for mental health and capability. Notwithstanding further developed cerebrum well-being, these unsaturated fats have been related to bringing down the gamble of coronary illness and joint inflammation. Salmon can be ready in different ways. It tends to be signed and matched with a good serving of vegetables or added to your number one pasta dish.

Our five-star Pecan Rosemary Crusted Salmon will assist with supporting your omega-3 admission in a scrumptious manner.

5. <u>Blueberries</u>

While all berries are gainful for mental well-being, blueberries are at the first spot on the list. They contribute fundamental supplements to the body, including L-ascorbic acid, vitamin K, manganese, and phytonutrients. These supplements help to animate the progression of blood and oxygen in the cerebrum, bringing about superior focus. A recent report distributed in General Wellbeing Sustenance recommends that eating an eating regimen containing different vegetables and organic products, like blueberries, is related to a lower chance of being old enough related to mental disability, dementia, and Alzheimer's sickness.

There are numerous ways of partaking in this delectable natural product — take a stab at adding a modest bunch to your smoothie recipe or pureeing a couple of berries to make a heavenly blueberry chia jam.

6. <u>Pecans</u>

Nuts are an incredible expansion to any eating routine, yet the one that contributes most to cerebrum wellbeing is pecans. When contrasted with different nuts, pecans offer two times as numerous cell reinforcements. They contain a fantastic wellspring of alpha-linolenic corrosive (ALA), which is a plant-based omega-3 fundamental unsaturated fat that assists with balancing mental degradation by stifling irritation and oxidative pressure. Irritation and oxidative pressure have been connected to Alzheimer's infection and dementia. A recent report distributed in Supplements recommends that eating around 1 to 2 ounces of pecans each day can work on mental capability. Have a go at adding a serving of pecans to a generous plate of mixed greens or matching them with different cooked vegetables.

Hints to work on your Memory

Even though there are no assurances about forestalling cognitive decline or dementia, a few exercises could help. Consider seven straightforward ways of honing your memory. Furthermore, know when to find support for cognitive decline.

1. <u>Be dynamic and consistently</u>

Active work raises the bloodstream to the entire body, including the cerebrum.

For most solid grown-ups, the Branch of Wellbeing and Human Administrations suggests something like 150 minutes every even-day stretch of moderate high-impact movement, like energetic strolling, or 75 minutes per seven-day stretch of fiery vigorous action, like running. It's ideal assuming that this action is spread over time. On the off chance that you cannot deal with a full exercise, attempt two or three 10-minute strolls over the day.

2. <u>Remain intellectually dynamic</u>

Similarly, as actual work keeps your body in shape, exercises that connect with your psyche assist with keeping your mind in shape. Furthermore, those exercises could assist with forestalling some cognitive decline. Do crossword puzzles. Peruse. Mess around. Figure out how to play an instrument. Attempt another leisure activity. Volunteer at a nearby school or with a local gathering.

3. Invest energy with others

Social connection helps avert sorrow and stress. Both of those can add to cognitive decline. Look for opportunities to coexist with loved ones, friends, and others, especially accepting you live alone.

4. Remain coordinated

You're bound to fail to remember things assuming your house is jumbled or your notes are in chaos. Monitor undertakings, arrangements, and different occasions in a scratch pad, schedule, or electronic organizer. You could try and rehash every passage without holding back as you record it to assist with keeping it in your memory. Stay up with the latest. Verify things you've wrapped up. Keep your wallet, keys, glasses, and other fundamental things in a set spot in your home so they are not difficult to track down.

Limit interruptions. Try not to do such a large number of things without a moment's delay. Assuming you center around the data that you're attempting to recollect, you're bound to review it later. It likewise could assist with interfacing what you're attempting to recollect to a main tune or a natural saying or thought.

5. <u>Rest soundly</u>

Not getting sufficient rest has been connected to cognitive decline. So has anxiety endless rest that gets upset frequently. Focus on getting sufficient solid rest. Grown-ups ought to rest 7 to 9 hours a night consistently. In the case of wheezing upsets rest, plan to see your medical services supplier. Wheezing could be an indication of a rest problem, like rest apnea.

6. <u>Eat a solid eating regimen</u>

A solid eating regimen is great for your mind. Eat organic products, vegetables, and entire grains. Select low-fat protein bases, like fish, beans, and skinless poultry. What you drink additionally counts. An excessive amount of liquor can prompt disarray and cognitive decline.

7. <u>Oversee persistent medical issues</u>

Follow your medical services supplier's guidance for managing ailments, for example, hypertension, diabetes, despondency, hearing misfortune, and weight. The more you bargain with yourself, the better your memory is likely to be. Consistently audit the meds you take with your medical services supplier. A few prescriptions can influence memory.

<u>When to find support for cognitive decline</u>

Assuming you're stressed over cognitive decline, make a meeting with your medical care supplier. On the off chance that cognitive decline influences your capacity to do your day-to-day exercises, on the off chance that you notice your memory deteriorating, or on the other hand if a relative or companion is worried about your cognitive decline, getting help is especially significant.

At your appointment, your supplier presumably will do an actual test and check your memory and critical thought capacities. In some cases, different tests might be required as well. Treatment relies upon what's causing cognitive decline.

Methods for Losing Gut Fat and Carry on with a Better Life

Weight The Executives Watch Your Weight Heart Well-being Heart-Savvy Eating. Greater waistlines are associated with a higher bet of coronary sickness, diabetes, and, surprisingly, threatening development. Getting in shape, especially stomach fat, in a like manner further creates vein working and further fosters the best quality.

It's hard to target stomach fat unequivocally when you diet. In any case, getting thinner generally will assist with contracting your waistline; all the more critically, it will assist with decreasing the hazardous layer of instinctive fat, a kind of fat inside the stomach cavity that you can't see however that uplifts well-being gambles, says Kerry Stewart, Ed.D., overseer of Clinical and Exploration Physiology at Johns Hopkins.

This is the way to garnish down where it brings in the major disparity.

1. <u>Make a pass at controlling carbs as opposed to fats.</u>

At the point when Johns Hopkins scientists looked at the consequences for the core of getting in shape through a low-carb diet versus a low-fat eating routine for a considerable timeframe — each containing a comparative proportion of calories — those on a low-carb diet lost an ordinary of 10 pounds more than those on a low-fat eating routine — 28.9 pounds versus 18.7 pounds. An extra benefit of the low-carb diet is that it conveyed a more prominent weight decrease, Stewart says. With weight decrease, fat is reduced, yet there is in like manner habitually a lack of fit tissue (muscle), which isn't charming.

2. <u>Continue to move.</u>

Active work helps consume stomach fat. The practice appears to work off midsection fat specifically because it lessens flowing degrees of insulin which would somehow flag the body to hold tight to fat.

3. Lift loads.

Adding even moderate strength preparing to vigorous activity assists work with inclining bulk, which makes you consume more calories throughout the whole day, both very still and during exercise.

4. Turn into a name peruser.

Investigate brands.   Nutrition mixtures like seasoning, mayonnaise, sauces, and salad dressings frequently contain high standards of lard and gears of calories.

5. Get away from handled food varieties.

The fixings in bundled products and nibble food varieties are in many cases weighty on trans fats, added sugar, and added salt or sodium — three things that make it challenging to get in shape.

6. Center around how your garments fit more than perusing a scale.

That is a superior characteristic of progress. Estimated around, your waistline ought to be under 35 inches on the off chance that you're a lady or under 40 inches assuming that you're a man to lessen heart and diabetes gambles.

Spend time with wellbeing centered companions.

Research shows that you're more ready to eat better and exercise accepting your friends and family are doing similarly.

Insulin: A chemical made by the cells in your pancreas. Assuming you have diabetes and your pancreas can't make enough of this chemical, you might be recommended drugs to help your liver make more or make your muscles more delicate to the accessible insulin. On the off chance that these meds are adequate not, you might be recommended insulin shots.

Veins: The arrangement of adaptable cylinders conduits, vessels, and veins — that help blood through the body. Oxygen and enhancements are passed by hallways onto little, wobbly-walled vessels that feed them to cells and get waste material, including carbon dioxide. Vessels pass the misfortune to veins, which return the blood to the heart and lungs, where carbon dioxide is let out through your breath as you inhale.

Corridors: The veins that divert oxygen-rich blood from your heart for conveyance to all aspects of your body. Corridors seem to be slender cylinders or hoses. The walls are made of an intense external layer, a center layer of muscle, and a smooth internal wall that assists blood with streaming without any problem. The muscle layer grows and agrees to assist with the blooding moves.

Recuperating FOOD Fundamentals THAT Advance Injury Mending

What you eat assumes a huge part in how your body capabilities on an everyday premise. Many individuals, in any case, don't ponder what the food they eat means for their body's injury-mending process. Eating a decent eating regimen of recuperating food varieties can assist your body with mending all the more rapidly and successfully.

What Food Fundamentals Are Great For Wound Mending?

A solid eating routine is a fundamental piece of the riddle for wound mending and keeping up with your general well-being and prosperity. That implies you ought to adjust your eating regimen and include every single dietary fundamental, particularly:

- **Proteins**
- **Micronutrients (nutrients and minerals)**
- **Sound Fats**
- **Carbs**

• <u>Protein's Job in Injury Mending</u>

Protein is seemingly one of the main parts of any eating routine since it is utilized in essentially every capability of your body. With regards to wound mending, protein is utilized to fix tissues, assist with conveying oxygen all through the body, and assist with warding off diseases.

Protein Required for Wound Mending

How much protein is required each day is subject to the individual, yet for the most part, the typical non-dynamic male necessities 56 grams each day. The typical non-dynamic female requires to eat 46 grams of protein each day. Individuals with wounds and different sicknesses need to eat more protein every day to help with injury recuperating. You might consider tracking down an injury care expert to assist with deciding the ideal sum required for you to mend.

Amino Acids and Wound Mending

Amino acids assist with building protein and are utilized in each cell of our bodies. Numerous amino acids play a part in building and fixing tissues, which is vital in injury mending.

<u>Recuperating Food Containing Amino Acids</u>

Arginine is an amino corrosive that assists increment with the bloodstream and oxygen to the injury. This outcome in expanded collagen arrangement and diminished irritation. Food varieties high in arginine incorporate pumpkin seeds, milk, yogurt, and cheddar.

One more significant amino corrosive in recuperating is glutamine which animates collagen creation, controls nitrogen digestion, and supports the resistant framework. Recovering food assortments high in glutamine consolidate chicken, fish, cabbage, spinach, dairy food sources, tofu, lentils, and beans.

<u>Micronutrients and Wound Mending</u>

The micronutrients required for a sound eating routine incorporate nutrients and minerals. While your body needs a large number of micronutrients, research shows that zinc and nutrients An and C are among probably the most indispensable for wound recuperation. Every one of these micronutrients is crucial for the body's intrinsic recuperating cycles, and when you don't get enough, you might see that you begin to feel more desolate than expected. They additionally assist with the body's fiery reaction and assist with creating collagen.

Other noteworthy micronutrients that are basic to wound recovery consolidate magnesium, iron, copper, vitamin E, and vitamin B.

Recuperating Food Containing Micronutrients

While it is ideal to eat various food sources to guarantee you get every one of the supplements you want for wound mending, a few decent decisions include:

Food varieties high in minerals: clams, spinach, nuts, for example, cashews, vegetables like peanuts, dairy items, dark beans, lentils, bananas, and fish.

Food varieties high in nutrients: citrus organic products, ringer peppers, entire grains, eggs, dim mixed greens, fish, lean meats, salad greens, soybeans, almonds, yams, and milk.

Sugars and Wound Mending

At the point when certain individuals hear "starches", they naturally contemplate how carbs separate into sugars, like glucose. Notwithstanding, when part of a solid, adjusted diet, this glucose is invested to great energy. Glucose is changed over into adenosine triphosphate (ATP), a sort of cell energy, which is utilized in the recuperating system.

Fats are Additionally Fundamental for Wound Mending

Solid fats (like unsaturated fats, lipids, phospholipids, linoleic and arachidonic acids) assume fundamental parts in keeping up with the body and empowering legitimate injury mending. Research has shown that these solid fats are fundamental for tissue regrowth and cell digestion and help with irritation.

Mending Food Containing Sound Fats

Food sources with fats that can add to wound mending incorporate sleek fish, avocados, nuts, seeds, and eggs.

Imagine a scenario in which Recuperating Food varieties Are Insufficient for Your Injury Mending.

About sustenance, it's critical to comprehend that all that you consume will affect your body and its capabilities. Eating an even eating regimen guarantees that your body can work appropriately and continue to make the fundamental cells expected to assist with conveying oxygen all through the body. You might need to talk with an enrolled nutritionist or dietician on the off chance that you want assistance adjusting your eating regimen, particularly about wound recuperating.

Tragically, in some cases, people should go through severe eating routine limitations, which can fundamentally affect their injury-mending capacity. Basic medical issues (like diabetes) additionally influence the body's capacity to recuperate well. On the off chance that this is your case, you might look for an injury facility to assist you with conceiving an arrangement to return you once again to well-being.

<u>Hyperbaric Twisted Care Alongside Recuperating Food varieties Can Assist with mending Wounds</u>

A few people might experience issues adjusting the important supplements expected to assist with conveying oxygen where it needs to go. Hyperbaric wound care treatment conveys 100 percent oxygen to the body through inward breath and ingestion. This guarantees your body is getting the oxygen it necessities to assist with further developing your body's injury-recuperating capacities. At the point when utilized related to a sustenance plan, they can guarantee you are getting the ideal medical advantages to assist your body with mending.

On the off chance that you would like an injury care expert to assess your mending or you have inquiries concerning hyperbaric oxygen treatment (HBOT).